EXERCISE IN THE MANAGEMENT OF CORONARY HEART DISEASE

A Guide for the Practicing Physician

EXERCISE IN THE MANAGEMENT OF CORONARY HEART DISEASE

A Guide for the Practicing Physician

By

GERALD F. FLETCHER, M.D.
Director of Internal Medicine
Georgia Baptist Hospital-Atlanta Medical Center
Assistant Professor of Medicine
Emory University School of Medicine
Atlanta, Georgia

and

JOHN D. CANTWELL, M.D.
Fellow in Medicine (Cardiology)
Emory University School of Medicine
Special Consultant to the Area Facility for Cardiovascular Disease
George Baptist Hospital-Atlanta Medical Center
Atlanta, Georgia

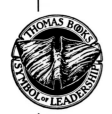

CHARLES C THOMAS · PUBLISHER
Springfiield · Illinois · U.S.A.

Published and Distributed Throughout the World by
CHARLES C THOMAS · PUBLISHER
BANNERSTONE HOUSE
301-327 East Lawrence Avenue, Springfield, Illinois, U.S.A.
NATCHEZ PLANTATION HOUSE
735 North Atlantic Boulevard, Fort Lauderdale, Florida, U.S.A.

With THOMAS BOOKS *careful attention is given to all details of
manufacturing and design. It is the Publisher's desire to present books
that are satisfactory as to their physical qualities and artistic possibilities
and appropriate for their particular use.* THOMAS BOOKS *will be true
to those laws of quality that assure a good name and good will.*

Printed in the United States of America
H-13

To my wife and children, for their mental and physical vigor and zest for an active, healthy life.

G.F.F.

To my parents, A.A.C., M.D., and A.D.C., who encouraged athletic participation and physical fitness as a way of life.

J.D.C.

PREFACE

C oronary atherosclerotic heart disease (herein referred to as coronary heart disease) is pandemic in the United States, claiming the lives of over 700,000 persons annually. It alone is the cause of 40 percent of all deaths. It is largely due to the frequent occurrence of coronary heart disease that our men rank eighteenth on a worldwide list of life expectancy. Coronary disease develops early in life, as evidenced by autopsy studies on American men killed in the Korean War,[1] British pilots killed in air crashes,[2] and Chilean men and women who died in automobile accidents.[3]

It is obvious that something must be done about this disease. Our current efforts are largely divided into three categories—prevention, diagnosis and treatment. The purpose of this book is to consider the role of exercise and physical training in these three areas. For years, exercise has either been overstated or underrated; it becomes necessary to separate facts from fads.

In the area of coronary disease prevention we will identify the more significant coronary risk factors and consider the effect of exercise training on each factor. In terms of the diagnosis of coronary disease, we will review the use of exercise stress testing and present data on a new method of exercise testing that is applicable to patients who are either at high coronary risk or who already show manifestations of the disease. Lastly, we will consider the use of exercise as a therapeutic agent in coronary heart disease and will outline a specific exercise program for the coronary patient. We will summarize the results of other investigators who have prescribed exercise for such patients and detail the hemodynamic findings as well as the risks and complications involved.

It is our hope that this book will be of particular use to the practicing physician, for it is he to whom the patient turns for scientific advice regarding exercise, it is he who will need to supervise the exercise if it is to be done properly, and it is he who will share in the ultimate consequences.

ACKNOWLEDGMENTS

WE WOULD LIKE to express our gratitude to Mary Peeples, R.N. for her editorial assistance and typing and to Mr. Howard Winters for his photography and art work in Figures 1, 2, 4-25, 27, 29 and 30.

CONTENTS

EXERCISE IN THE MANAGEMENT OF CORONARY HEART DISEASE

A Guide for the Practicing Physician

I

INTRODUCTION

$$\sim\sim\sim\sim\sim\sim\sim\sim\sim\sim\sim\sim\sim\sim\sim\sim\sim\sim\sim\sim\sim\sim\sim\sim\sim\sim\sim\sim\sim$$

THE ARCHIVES OF ancient history, as early as the time of Plato, have referred to the effects of exercise. Timaeus spoke of the body: "by moderate exercise reduces to order according to their affinities the particles and affections which are wandering about."[4] Richard Steele (1672-1729) stated that "reading is to the mind what exercise is to the body."[5]

Exercise, as an adjunct to good physical health, attained popularity early in American history. In 1785, Thomas Jefferson, while minister to France, wrote to his nephew: "Walking is the best possible exercise. Habituate yourself to walk fast without fatigue."[6] In 1854, concerning treatment of fatty degeneration of the heart, Stokes said that a person must adapt early hours and graduated exercise.[4]

During his influential years Doctor Paul White[7] has referred to our modern easy way of living as a "real pity"—he feels that our ancestors were in better physical health because of their active lives spent in clearing the forests and plowing the land. He feels that exercise is the "best tranquilizer there is." In farewell comments to his many friends and acquaintances he is known to never say "take it easy" but rather to say "take it hard."

Over the years it has been generally accepted that those persons who have physically active occupations enjoy better physical health; such an assumption, however, is not totally supported by sound evidence. Isolated case histories such as that of Clarence DeMar,[8] the marathon runner of the early 1900's, provide striking examples of the benefits of long-term physical conditioning. DeMar participated in marathon races for forty-nine years, and at his death (of metastatic rectal cancer) at age seventy, his coronary arteries at autopsy were two to three times the normal diameter.

Although much evidence supports the benefits of exercise in patients with coronary heart disease, its role continues to be somewhat controversial to practicing physicians. Complications such as sudden death occurring in joggers have kindled this controversy. In this book, we will consider several aspects of exercise—the advantages, the disadvantages, and the complications and risks. A discussion of proper exercise and comments on the use of exercise in the evaluation, prevention and therapy of coronary heart disease will be included in an attempt to clarify aspects of this problem.

II

ADVANTAGES OF EXERCISE

~~~~~~

EXERCISE IS GENERALLY thought to enhance and improve many bodily functions. Katz et al.[9] state vividly that physical fitness results in greater vital capacity, improves ability to relax, and develops better muscular tone; with regard to the cardiovascular system, he describes increased stroke volume, increased velocity of ventricular contraction, decreased blood pressure, decreased heart rate and diminished peripheral vascular resistance in well-trained individuals.

More specifically, regarding the cardiovascular system, there is considerable supportive evidence that physical activity and exercise is beneficial. In 1953, Morris and associates[10] studied the conductors and the drivers of London buses; they found that the incidence of coronary heart disease was less frequent in the more physically active conductors than in the sedentary drivers. An associated observation revealed that postmen had a lesser incidence of coronary heart disease that that of their more sedentary colleagues. When analyzed with regard to mortality, it has been shown that among presumably more active persons sudden death is less likely.[11] In addition, in pathologic studies, Morris and Crawford[12] found that the more active individuals had fewer large fibrous patches, fewer small multiple scars and fewer large, healed infarctions.

In the United States a study of mortality data in California showed that sedentary workers had a 40 percent greater fatality from coronary heart disease than did heavy workers.[13] Frank et al.[14] also showed a striking association between physical inactivity and early mortality from the initial myocardial infarction in men less than sixty-five years of age. Thus, there is evidence in population studies that physically active people are less likely to develop coronary heart disease and its complications.

[5]

From another vantage point, we must consider experimental evidence such as that provided by Eckstein,[15] who studied the effect of exercise and coronary artery narrowing on coronary collateral circulation in dogs. He discovered that collateral flow was greater in the exercised animals. Several other investigators [16,17] also found that regular exercise stimulates growth of the coronary vascular tree. Kaplinsky *et al.*[18] failed to detect any augmentation of coronary collateral vessels in dogs with exercise training; however, this might have been related to the technique of complete ligation of a large coronary vessel. Thus some experimental evidence supports the benefits of exercise. Evidence in humans is confined to isolated reports in several subjects in which serial coronary angiograms before and after training showed suggestive widening of local stenotic atherosclerotic lesions.[19] However, one study mentioned by Frick[20] did not show this. One of Hellerstein's cases[21] failed to show this, and several in the Mayo Clinic study[22] showed no change.

Therefore, although there is considerable evidence to support the benefits of exercise and physical training in patients with coronary heart disease there are still many unanswered questions.

III

DISADVANTAGES, COMPLICATIONS AND RISKS OF EXERCISE

THE TRUE DISADVANTAGES of exercise are less well supported than the advantages; however, a variety of exercise complications—cardiac and noncardiac—have been reported. In 1966 Keys[23] reported in European population sample studies that the more physically active Finns have more coronary deaths than do American whites. Other similar studies[24] have shown little or no difference in coronary heart disease death rate among those various occupations involving different levels of physical activity in the Chicago area.

Regarding complications, the major factors to be concerned with are sudden death, myocardial infarction and arrhythmias. On occasions news media report the occurrence of sudden death in a subject while jogging; not infrequently, we hear authenticated verbal reports of such complications. These deaths are most likely due to myocardial infarction, arrhythmias or cerebral vascular accidents. With regard to myocardial infarction,[25] we have seen a typical example on a 44-year-old male who, after an idle, sedentary period of life of twenty years, began a YMCA "Run For Your Life" program. He was not thoroughly evaluated by a physician prior to exercise and did not have an electrocardiogram or other studies. Because of his poor physical condition, he did no more than mild calesthenics and walking for the first two weeks after which he still retained his muscular soreness. The next day he attempted to slowly jog a mile, had chest pain and was admitted to a hospital with an acute inferior myocardial infarction (Fig. 1). After an initial period of an atrioventricular junctional rhythm he did well and was discharged. An example of an apparent cardiac dysrhythmia has been seen in a

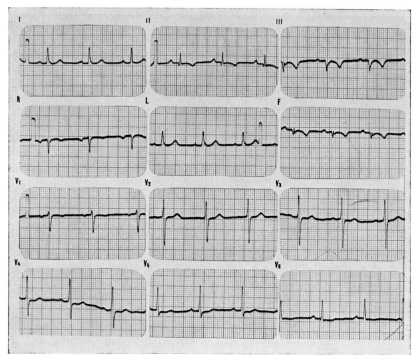

FIGURE 1. Twelve lead electrocardiogram of a 44-year-old male who had an acute inferior myocardial infarction while jogging. The abnormal Q waves and ST-T segments are seen in leads II, III and F.

middle-aged subject who collapsed while jogging and became cyanotic without pulse. He was successfully resusitated by a physician jogging behind him and treated successfully for a myocardial infarction.

Lesser or minor factors occurring during jogging and other types of exercise which tend to debilitate the exercise enthusiast or perhaps cause dropouts from exercise programs are not infrequently seen. Harris and Bowerman[26] reported seven subjects who developed acute gout in a group of 265 subjects who exercised. Other reported complications include development of petechiae,[27] "jogger's heel,"[28] exacerbations of osteoarthritis[29] and severe persistent muscular soreness which accounted for thirty-four of the ninety-eight dropouts reported by Harris and Bowerman.[26]

A recent evaluation in our laboratory of a group of twenty-three healthy male joggers who agreed to pretraining and post-training electrocardiograms and treadmill exercise testing revealed that five of the twenty-three subjects (22 percent) failed to return for retesting; of those retested seven had missed greater than ten of thirty-five training sessions. Ten subjects had abnormal resting electrocardiograms including an old myocardial infarction in one and frequent premature ventricular contractions (PVCs) in another. These subjects safely completed the jogging program, however, the latter developed "coupled" premature ventricular contractions during post-training exercise testing. In most subjects retested, neither heart rate nor maximal treadmill endurance changed significantly; none developed significant S-T changes or angina. This study revealed little data to support the physical benefits of jogging after a three-month period of training and illustrates some difficulties in such an evaluation. However, it is felt that a longer period of training might result in definite improvement; Mann *et al.*[30] found such improvement in their study after a six-month period. Another group of normals are now being evaluated on this basis in our laboratory; however, the value of screening such subjects for potential cardiovascular abnormalities is apparent even from the initial study.

Therefore, it is clear that physical training programs are interrupted at times by major and minor complications that are instrumental in preventing subjects from completing training programs. Further comments on the prevention of such complications and ways to make physical training more practical and efficient are forthcoming.

IV

THE HEMODYNAMICS OF PROPER EXERCISE

I n dealing with patients we, as physicians, are obligated to consider what goals we are trying to attain through exercise and what parameters we are trying to alter in the cardiovascular system.[31] These goals should be made clear when we discuss exercise with our patients.

The external stress that one may impose on the human body through some types of exercise may not actually alter the work of the heart itself or enhance "conditioning" of the cardiovascular system. For example, gardening, yard work and household domestic duties may impose extreme fatigue and musculoskeletal strain on a subject but do not necessarily cause high-caloric expenditure; to the contrary, jogging, swimming and brisk walking cause higher levels of caloric expenditure and are considered a more efficient type of exercise. The calories expended per hour for such various types of physical activity are listed in Figure 2 which data is taken in part from Falls.[32] Similar information is seen in Figure 3 relating the work classification scheme of Wells et al.[33]

In a direct consideration of the cardiovascular system what we must also consider in recommending exercise and evaluating exercise are those factors that determine the work done by the heart; that is, the myocardial oxygen consumption. Sarnoff et al.[34] and Monroe et al.[35] have clearly shown through physiological measures that myocardial oxygen consumption or heart work is directly related to the heart rate, systemic blood pressure or intraventricular pressures and the inotropic or contractile state of the myocardium. These principles have been transposed to the clinical setting most vividly in the work of Robinson.[36] He found in his group of fifteen patients with angina pectoris exposed to various types of progressive exercise and followed

[10]

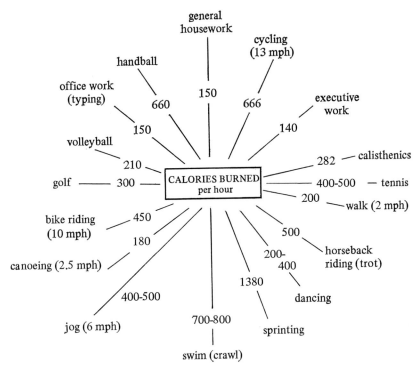

FIGURE 2. Chart showing the calories utilized per hour for various types of physical activity.

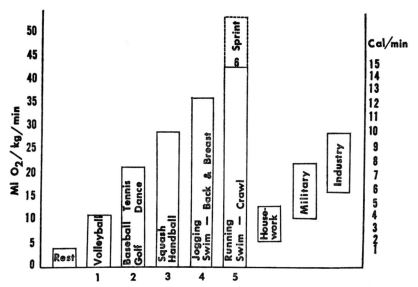

FIGURE 3. Bar graph showing oxygen consumption (milliliters per kilogram per minute) related to calories expended per minute for various levels of physical activity. The graph is from the work classification scheme of Wells et al.[22] with permission of Harold B. Falls, Ph.D., from the J. S. Carolina Med. Ass., 65:8, 1969.

with exercise testing that the threshold at which pain developed was always related to a fixed level of systolic blood pressure and heart rate. Regardless of the duration of the type of exercise, the work level of the heart that precipitated angina in each patient was always at the same level of pulse and blood pressure.

The circulatory dynamics of exercise have been of interest for many years. In 1957, Mitchell *et al.*[37] related evidence that maximal oxygen intake is a measure of cardiac capacity and the ability to increase the arteriovenous oxygen difference, not of the ability of the vascular bed to accomodate left ventricular output. Because of this they felt that maximal oxygen consumption had clinical usefulness in evaluating patients with cardiovascular disease. In 1963, Frick *et al.*[38] studied fourteen young men with sedentary habits. After a two-month hard training period they found that the subjects had an increase in heart volume, higher cardiac output at rest and reduced heart rate at rest in eleven of the fourteen subjects. During exercise, after training, these subjects had a larger stroke volume and a significantly lower heart rate. In 1968, Saltin *et al.*[39] studied five young normals extensively in a longitudinal study lasting three months. During the bed rest period of twenty days there was a pronounced decrease in maximal oxygen upstroke, stroke volume and cardiac output. At the end of a following fifty-five day training period, two previously trained subjects were able to attain the same level of maximal oxygen upstroke as they had reached in the initial control studies. Three previously sedentary subjects reached levels after training that were higher than their control values. In these latter three subjects the increase in maximal oxygen upstroke after training was attributable to increase in stroke volume and to widening of the arteriovenous oxygen difference. In addition to these aforementioned apparent hemodynamic benefits of training in normal young people, similar studies from the same laboratory by Siegel *et al.*[40] have shown a maximal oxygen uptake increase of 19 percent in nine healthy, blind sedentary men who participated in a fifteen-week quantitative physical training program.

Studies on older physically well-trained individuals have shown, in contrast to younger normals, that aerobic work capacity decreases with increasing age.[41] This is a basic principle to be aware of when testing individuals in the older age group especially because of their predilection to coronary disease.

Regarding studies in cardiovascular hemodynamics in patients with heart disease several authors have related their experiences. Naughton *et al.,*[42] in 1966, studied twenty-four men with well-documented myocardial infarctions; twelve participated in a physical conditioning program and the remainder remained sedentary. After eight months the trained cardiac patients had significant training effects as reflected by the systolic and diastolic blood pressure and pulse rate during rest, standing and comparable levels of energy expenditures. The response of the cardiac patient to that of a group of healthy normals indicated that the presence of disease did not necessarily affect the physiologic response of the subject.

In 1966, Varnauskas *et al.*[43] investigated the hemodynamic and metabolic effects of physical training in nine patients with coronary disease. In addition to clinical improvement after training they reported a hemodynamic adjustment toward a hypokinetic state and reduction in work of the left ventricle. Later in 1968, Frick *et al.*[44] assessed the hemodynamic effects of physical training in seven patients after myocardial infarction. The training was followed by reduction in exercise heart rate and tension time index, enhanced stroke volume and improved left ventricular function. Concommitant with these hemodynamic changes exercise tolerance was improved.

In accordance with such clinical and hemodynamic observations, leaders in exercise programming are being urged to design their training programs to deal with the simple factors of blood pressure and heart rate; that is, to design training with the end point in mind of elevating the heart rate to a certain level in order to condition the heart. Figure 4 shows examples of various heart rates based on the data of Sheffield *et al.*[45] for given ages that are currently in use in training programs. These rates are depicted for the 70 and 85 percent of maximum heart rate (MHR) levels; it is felt that the 70% MHR is best used as an endpoint for exercise and the 85% MHR levels are best reserved for an exercise testing endpoint in the presence of a physician. Using these parameters through selected exercise over a long period of training (such as a jogging

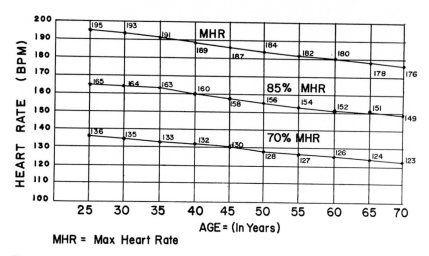

FIGURE 4. Graph showing various levels of heart rate in beats per minute (BPM) expressed as maximum heart rate, 85%, and 75% of maximum. The heart rate is plotted with age in years. The data is based on that of Sheffield *et al.*[45]

program) it has been shown that a person can achieve a progressively greater level of exercise with less acceleration of the heart rate,[46] thus reducing the work of the heart for a given level of exercise. Likewise, through such physical training, maximal blood pressure elevation can be decreased for the same level of exercise, again decreasing the work of the heart. Therefore, with this more scientific approach to exercise, more benefit can be achieved with less complications that are frequently associated with inefficient efforts.

V

EXERCISE TESTING IN EVALUATION OF HEART DISEASE – A DIAGNOSTIC TOOL

I̶N̶ EVALUATION OF heart disease, exercise testing with use of the step test, bicycle ergometer or a treadmill is of great value. As early as 1929, Master *et al.*[47] reported the use of the step test to evaluate subjects with coronary heart disease. Doan *et al.*,[48] in 1965, summarized the positivity of these tests in postexercise electrocardiograms in most males as ranging from 0 to 37.09 percent; the type testing used in these studies being double and single Master tests and bicycle ergometry. In contrast to these studies, the isolated Seattle study of normal males[48] revealed a much higher prevalence rate of 136 per 1,000 by clinical examination and treadmill exercise testing. Compared to the Albany study[49] in which moderate treadmill exercise testing was done, the minimal detection rate of positive tests using the Seattle method of multistage maximal treadmill exercise testing was 3.3 times higher. These tests were, of course, performed in normal individuals and the maximal test was felt to be a safe method of evaluation. The need for a well-defined exercise test for patients with coronary heart disease was illustrated in a recent report by Roitman *et al.*[50] They used the Bruce test for persons judged to have a "more normal" exercise capacity but followed an ill-defined and difficult-to-reproduce test for ones with overt coronary heart disease.

In our hands a submaximal treadmill exercise test has been of great value in the evaluation of patients with clinical evidence either diagnostic of or strongly suggestive of ischemic heart disease. This testing is done at a constant treadmill speed of two miles per hour (mph) beginning at zero percent grade and increasing the grade two and one-half percent every two and one-half minutes. Details of our testing procedure are seen in Table 1. It is felt that the constant speed

[15]

TABLE 1
STAGES OF SUBMAXIMAL TREADMILL EXERCISE TEST

Stage	Speed (mph)	Elevation (%)	Time (min.)
1	2	0	2½
2	2	2½	2½
3	2	5	2½
4	2	7½	2½
5	2	10	2½
6	2	12½	2½
7	2	15	2½
8	2	17½	2½
9	2	20	2½
10	2	22½	2½

with increasing slope poses less external muscular stress on the subject, but instead, a gradual stress to the cardiovascular system and thus is a more reliable evaluation of circulatory response.

Patients evaluated were both outpatients and inpatients referred by their respective physicians for submaximal treadmill exercise testing. Specific reasons for referral included chest pain, arrhythmias, syncope or clinical suspicion of heart disease (based on a high incidence of risk factors) in a patient about to begin a physical training program. None of these patients were on digitalis or beta adrenergic blocking agents. A constant speed, variable grade treadmill test was used with continuous direct electrocardiographic monitoring. The monitoring was done with a two lead bipolar chest electrode system producing a simulated V5. The signal was viewed constantly on the oscilloscope with intermittent graphic write out on a standard electrocardiogram machine. Figure 5 shows the equipment used in testing. Blood pressure was monitored by cuff sphygmomanometer. A direct current defibrillator, as well as emergency cardiac drugs, were available in the room and a physician and registered nurse were in attendance for all testing.

The protocol for exercise evaluation began with clear explanation to the patient by the physician and nurse as to the nature of the testing and what was expected of the patient. A twelve lead standard electrocardiogram was recorded before the test. Electrodes were then secured to the chest with electrode paste and adhesive pads with the patient in a chair on the side platform of the treadmill. A cuff sphygmomanometer was placed on the upper arm and a baseline blood

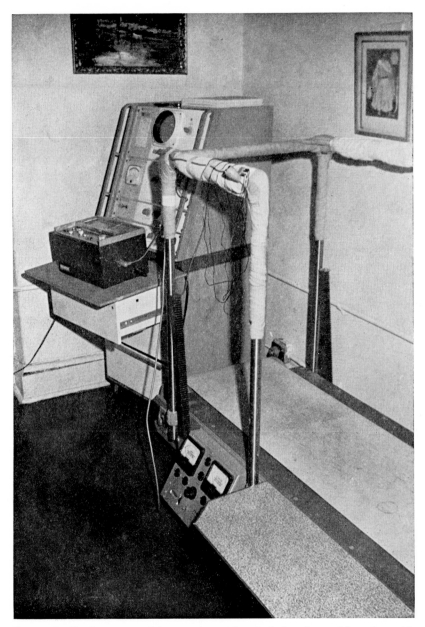

FIGURE 5. Equipment used in exercise testing includes the multispeed, multigrade treadmill, with direct wire electrodes for chest lead monitoring. In the background near the treadmill is a direct current defibrillator with oscilloscope for constant visual electrocardiographic monitoring. The direct writing electrocardiogram machine is used for intermittent permanent recordings.

pressure was recorded. A sample electrocardiographic tracing was recorded to assure a clear recording for purposes of evaluating heart rate, rhythm, and S-T segment displacement.

The treadmill exercise evaluation was begun with the patient in the standing position at which time a baseline electrocardiogram recording was made. The treadmill was then turned on for the beginning of stage one (0% elevation at 2 mph) at which time the patient was instructed to accustom himself to the motion of the treadmill by walking with his right foot on the belt while maintaining his balance and weight on the other stationary extremity. After becoming accustomed to the motion the subject was instructed to begin walking on the belt. At this point the timing for stage one was begun with a stopwatch. Patients were instructed to walk erect, look ahead, and to maintain balance by lightly gripping the side rail.

The exercise was continued through the stages outlined in Table 1 with a constant speed of 2 mph with elevation of the slope by $2\frac{1}{2}$ percent every two and one-half minutes. The electrocardiogram recordings of a simulated V5 was constantly observed on the oscilloscope and a graphic record of 8 to 10 cycles was made at one-minute intervals. In the event of an arrhythmia being seen on the oscilloscope, additional written recordings were made. In addition to the constant electrocardiogram recordings, blood pressure was recorded by auscultation every three minutes.

The patients were urged to walk to the point of moderate to severe fatigue or dyspnea or to the point of anginal-type pain. Other limiting factors included heart rate elevation of approximately 85 percent of the maximal expected rate for the patients age. Development of arrhythmias or significant S-T segment displacement of one or more millimeters for .08 second duration as well as blood pressure elevation of 240 mm Hg (systolic) or more also constituted criteria for termination of the test. The physician and nurse were in constant communication with the patient and the patients were urged to describe even the slightest functional and/or physical symptoms that developed as the testing progressed.

At the termination of the test the subject was instructed to sit in a chair on the treadmill while immediate, one, two and three minute postexercise rhythm strips and blood pressure recordings were made.

The subjects were observed closely for symptoms and signs of dizziness, near-syncope or postional hypotension; if such developed they were placed in a supine position until stable.

One hundred patients were evaluated in our laboratory with submaximal treadmill exercise testing over a period of eight months. The age range was from twenty-six to seventy-five years with an average age of 50.1 years. There were seventy-five male patients and twenty-five females. Only one subject was black (a forty-year-old female); the remainder were Caucasian. The range of duration of test time was 0.5 minutes to 26.0 minutes with an average of 10.7 minutes. The range of maximum heart rate attained was from 80 beats per minute to 180 beats per minute with an average for the group of 132 beats per minute.

TABLE 2
CUMULATIVE DATA ON 100 PATIENTS UNDERGOING
SUBMAXIMAL TREADMILL EXERCISE TESTING

	No. of Patients (100)	%
Positive S-T segment displacement		
Before angina	5	5
After angina	12	12
Development of/or increase in PVCs	13	13
Development of/or increase in PNCs	6	6
Development of/or increase in PACs	2	2
Blood pressure of 200 mm Hg or more systolic	4	4
Abnormal resting ECG	44	44
Abnormal resting ECG in patients with		
Positive exercise test	15 of 17	88.2
Normal exercise test	29 of 83	34.9
Positive exercise test in patients with		
Abnormal resting ECG	15 of 44	34.1
Normal resting ECG	2 of 56	3.6

PVCs—premature ventricular contractions; PNCs—premature nodal contractions; PACs—premature atrial contractions; ECG—electrocardiogram; mm Hg—millimeters of mercury.

A summary of the testing results are seen in Table 2. As noted, 17 percent of the patients (17 of 100) showed ischemic S-T segment changes. An example of such a patient is seen in Figure 6. Thirteen percent (13 of 100) had development of or increase in ventricular ectopic beats and 8 percent (8 of 100) developed supraventricular ectopic beats (premature atrial contractions and premature nodal contractions). Of this group of one hundred patients one (with (history of undocumented tachycardia) developed paroxysmal atrial

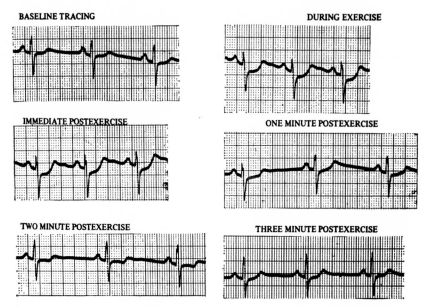

FIGURE 6. Submaximal treadmill exercise test results in a 62-year-old male with symptoms suggestive of angina pectoris. Positive S-T segment changes indicative of ischemic heart disease are best seen during (after four minutes of exercise) and immediately after exercise.

tachycardia (160 beats per minute) during exercise to document the arrhythmia (see Fig. 7). Another, with a previous supraventricular tachycardia that had required cardioversion, developed frequent premature ventricular contractions during exercise to further document a suspected abnormality to explain his tachyarrhythmia (see Fig. 8).

Analysis of the resting twelve lead electrocardiogram in the seventeen patients with positive tests for ischemic heart disease revealed that 88.2 percent (15 of 17) were abnormal—all of which had some degree of abnormality of the ST-T segments. In addition, four of these fifteen had evidence of old myocardial infarction on resting electrocardiogram. Analysis of the resting electrocardiograms of all the patients revealed that 44 percent (44 of 100) were abnormal; of these forty-four, the most common abnormality was ST-T changes which were seen in 50 percent (22 of 44). Of these forty-four with abnormal electrocardiograms 34.1 percent (15 of 44) had positive tests for ischemic heart disease.

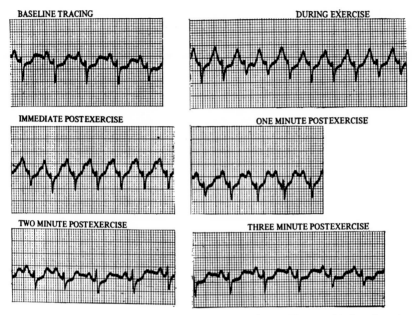

FIGURE 7. Submaximal treadmill exercise test in a 42-year-old female who developed paroxysmal atrial tachycardia (160 beats per minute) at the eleven-minute level during exercise. The patient became dizzy, had near-syncope and the test was terminated at this point.

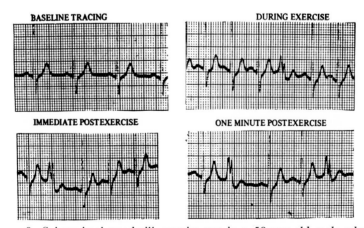

FIGURE 8. Submaximal treadmill exercise test in a 58-year-old male who developed frequent premature ventricular contractions at eight minutes of exercise. This aided in documenting a suspected abnormality to explain a previously reported tachyarrhythmia.

No one in the group developed a hypertensive crisis (above 240 mm Hg systolic elevation) and no syncope or extreme dizziness developed in anyone. No one fell although one emotionally labile subject stepped off the treadmill unexpectedly. The postexercise recovery periods were uneventful; no one developed hypotension although several of the patients who developed ischemic changes or arrhymias had these persist through part of the recovery period.

In general, the results of our treadmill exercise evaluation program for subjects with heart disease have been revealing to us and helpful to the private physician caring for the patient.

VI

EXERCISE IN PREVENTION OF
CORONARY HEART DISEASE
EFFECT ON THE RISK FACTORS

$\sim\sim\sim\sim\sim\sim\sim\sim\sim\sim\sim\sim\sim\sim\sim\sim\sim\sim\sim\sim\sim\sim\sim\sim\sim\sim$

Numerous studies[51-55] have led to the identification of multiple factors which seem to predispose one to coronary heart disease. A cross-sampling of several such studies produces the following list of the more frequently implicated coronary risk factors:

1. Blood lipid abnormalities
2. Hypertension
3. Cigarette smoking
4. Carbohydrate intolerance
5. Physical inactivity
6. Overweight
7. Diet
8. Heredity
9. Personality and behavior patterns
10. Electrocardiographic abnormalities
11. Disorders in blood coagulation
12. Elevation in blood uric acid.
13. Pulmonary function abnormalities

It is difficult to assess the relative importance of each factor in comparison to the others, although a recent report[56] placed greater emphasis on blood pressure and cholesterol. Many of the factors are interrelated, such as blood lipid abnormalities, diabetes, heredity, and obesity. Individual studies taken alone can contribute to this confusion. For example, one can compare the relative importance of diet and physical inactivity: Irish men residing in their native country consumed more calories and saturated fat than did their

[23]

blood brothers residing in the United States[57]; yet, they had a significantly lesser incidence of coronary heart disease. The latter was felt by some to reflect their increased physical activity, which was mainly in the form of bicycle riding and manual labor. Exercise might also be the reason why the Masai tribesmen of East Africa have such a low incidence of atherosclerosis despite eating foods extremely high in saturated fats.[58] Other studies have indicated that regular exercise is certainly no panacea against premature coronary disease. The Rendille tribesmen of Africa exercise vigorously each day but consume a diet high in saturated fat and have a high incidence of atherosclerosis.[59] An evaluation of risk factors in young prisoners with premature myocardial infarctions (prior to age thirty-nine) revealed that four men had exercised vigorously on a daily basis for up to three years prior to the attack.[60] One such individual jogged from two to five miles per day. A recent report[61] compared one hundred male military personnel who survived a myocardial infarction at age forty or less with a control group. There was no significant difference in physical activity between the two groups. Such reports can be misleading in that the accustomed degree of physical activity was determined by questionnaires rather than by direct interrogation.

Despite the deficiencies in the analysis of risk factors, they remain the most reliable simple screening device that we have available at present. It is therefore worthwhile to review the effect of exercise on the respective factors for this might serve as an objective means of explaining the subjective improvements most physically fit persons profess. To do this, let us take the previously mentioned thirteen risk factors on an individual basis.

1. Blood Lipid Abnormalities

Lipoprotein electrophoresis techniques have enhanced our knowledge of the different types of hyperlipidemias.[62] Despite such sophisticated techniques, the serum cholesterol and triglyceride levels remain the most practical screening tests. Decreases in serum cholesterol following an active physical conditioning program have been noted by many investigators. These include studies on prisoners,[63] army officers,[64] postcoronary patients,[65-66] and the general population.[30] The latter study indicated that the amount of decrease was related to the percentage of exercise sessions attended over a six-month period. The duration of individual exercise sessions and of the total physical conditioning period was quite variable. Siegel *et al.*[40] reported a mean decrease in serum cholesterol from 247 to 210 mg% in nine blind men who were exercised for only twelve minutes three times per week over a fifteen-week period. This was independent of any weight change. On the other hand, despite sixteen hours of vigorous daily physical activity over a twenty-two week period, there was no significant decrease in the serum cholesterol of 101 marine trainees.[67] Others have reported similar experience.[68,69,70] Holloszy *et al.*[68] studied twenty-seven subjects over a six-month period of vigorous training and found no change in serum cholesterol nor in serum phospholipids. Studies comparing cross-country skiers[71] and college athletes[68] with age-matched non-athletes detected no difference in cholesterol levels.

It appears then that there is no uniform agreement as to whether exercise per se has a significant effect on the serum cholesterol level. Many of the preceeding studies are difficult to interpret because true control groups were not mentioned, seasonal variations in lipid levels were not considered, and details of concomitant weight and dietary alterations are lacking.[72-73] Furthermore, Mirkin[74] pointed out a marked lability in serum cholesterol on a day-to-day basis during a long-distance running program.

In the well-controlled study by Holloszy *et al.*[68] six months of physical training resulted in a significant decrease in serum triglycerides (from a mean of 208 mg% to a mean of 125 mg%) in fourteen men. This change, however, was found to persist for only approximately two days following each exercise session. Nikkila and Konttinen[75] found a similar decrease in triglycerides after acute exercise in one group, but no such changes in a control group. The usual postprandial increase in triglycerides was appreciably reduced by exercise in the group studied by Cohen *et al.*[76] Hoffman *et al.*[64] reported a triglyceride-lowering response to exercise but furnished no information concerning weight change and comparison with a control group. Several reports suggest either no change[43,68,77] or an increase in serum triglyceride levels following physical training.[30,67] This probably can be explained by an accompanying increase in food intake. Although Siegel *et al.*[40] found a mean decrease in serum triglyceride of 137 to

82 mg%, they did not feel this to be of significance. They made no mention as to how long postexercise the samples were collected.

Thus, exercise seems to have a transient lowering effect on post-exercise and postprandial triglyceride levels. This might serve as an indicator for the frequency of exercise sessions (every forty-eight hours at least). The elevations in serum triglycerides during exercise training are most likely related to dietary alterations.

2. Hypertension

Considerable data has accumulated to indicate a modest blood pressure-lowering effect of exercise, [4,12,38,78,79] both in normals[26] and in postcoronary patients.[66] Mann et al.[30] found a decrease in both systolic and diastolic levels as did Boyer and Kasch[80] and Naughton et al.,[42] and all three studies featured control groups. Mellerowicz[81] noted that trained sportsmen had an average systolic blood pressure 20 mm Hg lower than the control group. Although Clausen et al.[65] found a significant decrease in systolic blood pressure in nine cardiac patients who underwent four to six weeks of physical training, other investigators have reported no basic change in arterial pressure.[43,44,67]

The evidence to date suggests that exercise therapy can produce reduction in both systolic and diastolic pressure in both hypertensive and normotensive persons. Similar changes probably occur in coronary patients, although additional data is needed.

3. Cigarette Smoking

According to the review by Fox and Skinner,[4] no adequate investigations have been conducted to determine whether physical exercise diminishes the desire for cigarette smoking. Such studies would indeed be difficult to substantiate, being primarily a subjective finding.

4. Carbohydrate Intolerance

In 1924, Levine et al.[82] reported that physical exercise was usually accompanied by a fall in the blood sugar level. In 1945, Blotner[83] noted improvement of glucose tolerance after exercise. Despite reports by Davidson et al.[84] that very intense physical training impairs glucose tolerance (based on only five subjects), clinical experience indicated that diabetics require less insulin when more physically active. Well-controlled studies, however, on physical training and insulin requirements are lacking. Nevertheless, Mann et al.[30] showed that the fasting blood sugar level could be significantly decreased after a six-month exercise program (involving sixty-two men), however the glucose tolerance did not change. There was no change in the fasting blood sugars of exercising cardiac patients, according to Frick and Katila,[44] but the group was small (seven men) and the frequency (three times per week) and duration of physical training (one to two months) were mild.

5 and 6. Physical Inactivity — Overweight

Significant weight loss in normal and obese persons has been noted in response to prolonged physical training.[20,26,30,85,86] Analysis of studies reporting no change or a weight gain during exercise therapy frequently reveal appreciable increases in caloric intake.[10] Perhaps the most representative study is that by Mann et al.[30] wherein a small but significant weight loss and loss of subcutaneous fat was recorded in the exercise group but not in the dropouts or controls. Regarding cardiac patients in exercise programs, Naughton et al.[42] found no weight change over an eight-month period of observation, although Hellerstein[66] recorded an average weight reduction of five pounds in a total of one hundred and fifty-eight men over a longer follow-up period (thirty-three months).

7, 8 and 9. Diet — Heredity —
Personality and Behavior Patterns

Although exercise per se has no direct effect on the type of diet that is consumed or on hereditary factors, it has been shown to cause changes in personality and behavior patterns.[87] Most of the latter changes are subjective, however. Nonetheless, in addition to a lessening of fatigue and an improvement in sleeping ability, Hellerstein[21] was able to measure an improvement in the depression scale on the Minnesota Multiphasic Personality Inventory (MMPI) in exercised cardiac patients. Naughton et al.[88] found no significant change in the MMPI in a smaller group but also noted the subjective improvements in sleep patterns and stress relationships. Hellerstein and Friedman,[89,90] in addition, found that improved physical fitness had a favorable effect on sexual activity in postcoronary patients. An increase in sexual tension, along with anxiety and alterations in sleep patterns, was found in fourteen college students during a thirty-day period of exercise deprivation.[91]

10. Electrocardiographic Abnormalities

Electrocardiographic abnormalities, namely voltage criteria for left ventricular hypertrophy[53] and premature ventricular contractions,[92] are additional coronary risk factors. Persons with left ventricular hypertrophy have an increased risk of death during an initial episode of myocardial infraction than do those without this finding.[93]

Strenuous physical activity may actually result in voltage criteria for left ventricular hypertrophy. Of twenty-one marathon runners studied, sixteen had voltage criteria suggesting this diagnosis.[94] While the hypertrophied ventricle of cardiac patients is felt to operate on a depressed Frank-Starling curve this does not seem to apply to the hypertrophy of exercise.[95] On the other hand, Hellerstein *et al.*[96] were able to show a disappearance of premature ventricular contractions in four persons who underwent physical conditioning.

11. Disorders In Blood Coagulation

Blood clotting alterations have been cited by several investigators. Although unaccustomed strenuous exercise can actually result in increased blood clotting and thrombus formation,[97,98] regular exercise in general prolongs blood clotting due to enhanced fibrinolysis.[97,99,100] Other risk factors can interact; for instance, hyperlipemia has been shown to accelerate blood clotting.[101,102] Additional studies of a significant number of patients and controls are warranted to further assess the interesting relationship between exercise and coagulation.

12. Elevations In Blood Uric Acid

Mann *et al.*[30] noted an increase in blood uric acid in exercising individuals. This may account for the cases of gout which developed for the first time in seven persons exercising under the supervision of Harris *et al.*[26]. Mann *et al.*[30] postulated that episodic hyperlactemia might interfere with urate excretion.

Although Montoye *et al.*[103] found that high school athletes had significantly higher serum uric acid levels than nonathletes, these levels tended to decrease during the active season of the particular athlete. This suggested a possible beneficial effect of exercise. Bosco *et al.*[104] revealed that serum uric acid levels were reduced from 0.3 to 3.2 mg/100 in 80 percent of twenty men who exercised over an eight-week period. The decrease was greatest in those with the highest initial serum uric acid levels and in those who underwent the most strenuous exercise. Calvy *et al.*[67] were unable to detect any significant changes in serum uric acid in Marine Corp recruits. More data is obviously needed to settle the relationship between exercise and uric acid.

13. Pulmonary Function Abnormalities

A decreased vital capacity as a coronary risk factor was noted in the Framingham Study.[105] Rechnitzer *et al.*[106] demonstrated an average increase in vital capacity of 570 cc in four coronary patients who exercised over a twelve-week period. No changes in vital capacity or in forced expiratory volumes were seen in sixteen other postcoronary patients,[44,65] although the duration of physical training was not as long (four to eight weeks). Exercise training was recently reported as promising in patients with chronic obstructive pulmonary disease.[107]

A summary of the present knowledge concerning the effects of exercise on the coronary risk factors can be seen in Table 3. Beneficial effects are indicated with plus $(+)$, adverse effects with minus $(-)$, and no effect with (NE). In other instances exercise is either unrelated (u) to the factor or there is insufficient evidence (IE) to indicate a positive or negative effect.

TABLE 3
EFFECTS OF EXERCISE ON CORONARY RISK FACTORS

Risk Factor	*Effect of Exercise*
1. Blood lipids	
a. Cholesterol	IE
b. Triglycerides	+
2. Blood pressure	
a. Systolic	+
b. Diastolic	+
3. Cigarette smoking	u
4. Blood sugar	
a. Fasting blood sugar	+
b. Glucose tolerance test	NE
5. Physical inactivity	+
6. Overweight	+
7. Diet	u
8. Heredity	u
9. Personality and behavior patterns	IE
10. EKG abnormalitites	
a. Premature ventricular contractions	+
b. Left ventricular hypertrophy	—
11. Blood clotting	IE
12. Blood uric acid	IE
13. Pulmonary function	
a. Vital capacity	IE
b. Forced expiratory volume	IE

+ = beneficial effects; u = unrelated; IE = insufficient evidence;
NE = no effect; — = adverse effects.

VII

EXERCISE THERAPY FOR CORONARY DISEASE
– A PRESCRIPTION

Recognition that exercise may be of benefit in treating coronary disease dates back to the initial description of angina pectoris. In 1772, Heberden[108] wrote that one of his patients was "nearly cured" of the disorder after sawing wood for thirty minutes daily over a six-month period. Seven years later, Parry[109] observed that foot soldiers rarely developed exertional heart disease and that perhaps their routine physical activity guarded against this.

Over the past decade numerous investigators have expounded the benefits of increased activity and regular exercise for angina pectoris and the postmyocardial infarction state. The studies dealing with the largest number of patients are those of Hellerstein[21] and Gottheimer.[110] The latter reported a five-year follow-up on 1,103 male patients with coronary disease, 548 of whom had a previous myocardial infarction (although criteria for diagnosis were not listed). The exercise program began with several months of mild strength-building activities, which included weight lifting. Specifics of this initial program are not provided. After about nine months, the men engaged in rhythmic endurance exercises such as running, hiking, swimming, cycling, rowing and volleyball. Those who excelled in these activities and achieved a significant improvement in overall fitness then entered competitive team games. The participants in the general exercise program basically practiced on their own on a twice-daily schedule. There was obviously no medical supervision. Once a week, the men met as a group for instructions and practice. The most impressive results of the study are in the mortality rate data which was 3.6 percent for the entire group over the five-year period in contrast to 12 percent of a comparable nonexercised group of Israeli with previous myocardial infarctions. Gottheimer described other objective effects of training, such as reductions of resting heart rate and of resting and exercise blood pressure levels. In addition, there was less S-T segment depression on electrocardiograms taken during and immediately after exercise. Unfortunately, the complete date on these observations is not given, which makes the significance questionable. Hellerstein[66] recently noted the results of physical training on 656 middle-aged males, 203 of whom had angina pectoris and/or myocardial infarction. An additional fifty-one men had resting or exercise stress test electrocardiograms compatible with silent coronary heart disease (utilizing the Minnesota Code). Persons with vascular disease and uncompensated congestive heart failure were excluded from the program. The coronary patients were followed for an average of 2.7 years. They participated in at least a thrice-weekly exercise program which consisted of calisthenics, run-walk sequences, and recreational activities. The latter included swimming, basketball, volleyball, and use of a punching bag. Detailed results were presented on the first one hundred cardiac patients. The average weight loss was 2.5 kg. Sixty-five percent significantly improved their level of fitness, as measured by bicycle ergometric testing and oxygen consumption. Sixty-three percent showed improvement in their exercise electrocardiograms, mainly in terms of the initial slope and the junctional displacement of the S-T segment. The death rate for the exercising cardiac patients was 1.9 per 100 patient years which was less than half the expected rate.

A wide variety of exercise programs have been utilized by the various investigators. Unfortunately, none are clearly and concisely outlined in the literature. In view of this, a modified regimen that was originally devised for a pilot project at the Mayo Clinic by one of the authors (JDC) and Mr. Edward Koch, a physical fitness director, is presented in detail. The program was tailored specifically for the postcoronary patient and can be modified according to the available laboratory facilities. In addition to the Mayo Clinic Study, this exercise regimen is being used in ongoing studies at Georgia Baptist Hospital-Atlanta Medical Center. The fundamentals of the program are as follows:

1. Patients must be at least three months postmyocardial infarction. They must be less than sixty-five years of age. Concomitant diseases such as uncompensated congestive heart failure, severe hypertension (diastolic blood pressure greater than 120 mm Hg), cardiac rhythm disturbances (such as frequent PVCs, paroxysms of tachycardia), vascular disease, and chronic lung disease prohibit inclusion into the program.

2. A minimum of three exercise sessions, each forty-five minutes in duration, are conducted weekly at a YMCA, local high school, or community recreation center. A physician is always in attendance. Resuscitation equipment including a portable electrocardiograph machine, direct current defibrillator and emergency drug kit are on hand. The forty-five minute sessions are divided into three fifteen-minute periods. The first consists of calisthenics, the second of walk-jog activity and the third of noncompetitive group activity such as volleyball, basketball and swimming. A five-minute warm-up period and a similar cool-down period is part of each session.

3. Patients are given an exercise prescription at the beginning of each week indicating the calisthenic and walk-jog activity for that week. The prescription is based on three factors: (a) direct participant observation by the physician in attendance, who frequently exercises with the patients; (b) preliminary and follow-up data, based on treadmill performance and oxygen consumption; and (c) the patient's subjective response to the given level of exercise (in terms of musculo-skeletal side effects and respiratory effort).

The calisthenics are conducted in five different positions and are designed to exercise the major muscle groups. Initially, the number of repetitions is low to avoid undue muscular strain and discouragement to the participant. After the initial six months, the number of repetitions are increased to the point where the individual is averaging 70 percent of his maximum pulse rate during the actual exercises. This requires radiotelemetry recording during the calisthenic period, when available, or a manual check of the pulse rate midway during each calisthenic position. The number of repetitions for a given week (for the first six months of exercise) are listed in the following chart with illustrations of each exercise as seen in Figures 9 through 25.

CORONARY GROUP EXERCISE CHART
Standing Position

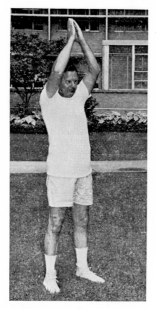

FIGURE 9. ARM AND SHOULDER LOOSENING
With subject in standing position the arms are raised overhead, bringing the palms together; the arms are then lowered to the sides, completing the sequence.

Week	Repetitions per session	Week	Repetitions per session
1	6	13	18
2	6	14	18
3	8	15	18
4	8	16	18
5	10	17	18
6	10	18	18
7	12	19	20
8	12	20	20
9	14	21	20
10	14	22	20
11	16	23	20
12	16	24	20

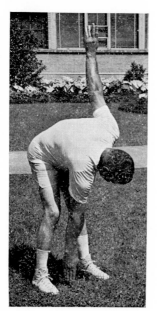

FIGURE 10. TOE TOUCHING

Keeping the knees straight, the subject flexes at the waist and touches the right fingertips to the left toes. He assumes an erect position and then touches the left fingertips to the right toes, completing the sequence.

Week	Repetitions per session	Week	Repetitions per session
1	4	13	12
2	4	14	12
3	5	15	12
4	5	16	12
5	6	17	12
6	6	18	12
7	8	19	14
8	8	20	14
9	10	21	14
10	10	22	14
11	12	23	14
12	12	24	14

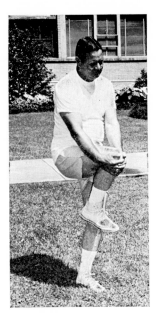

✓ FIGURE 11. KNEE RAISING

The subject grasps the left knee with both hands and raises it as high as he can. He then does the same thing to the right knee, completing one cycle.

Week	Repetitions per session	Week	Repetitions per session
1	6	13	14
2	6	14	14
3	7	15	14
4	7	16	14
5	8	17	14
6	8	18	14
7	10	19	16
8	10	20	16
9	12	21	16
10	12	22	16
11	14	23	16
12	14	24	16

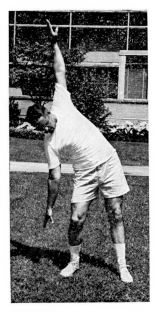

✓ FIGURE 12. LATERAL BENDING

With the arms elevated in a horizontal position the subject bends laterally to the left, assumes an erect position and then bends laterally to the right.

Week	Repetitions per session	Week	Repetitions per session
1	4	13	12
2	4	14	12
3	5	15	12
4	5	16	12
5	6	17	12
6	6	18	12
7	8	19	14
8	8	20	14
9	10	21	14
10	10	22	14
11	12	23	14
12	12	24	14

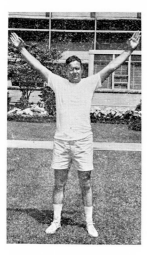

✓FIGURE 13. ARM CIRCLING

The arms are elevated in a horizontal position
and rotated, first clockwise for the given number
of repetitions and then counterclockwise for the
same number of times.

Week	Repetitions per session	Week	Repetitions per session
1	8	13	14
2	8	14	14
3	10	15	14
4	10	16	14
5	10	17	14
6	10	18	14
7	12	19	16
8	12	20	16
9	12	21	16
10	12	22	16
11	14	23	16
12	14	24	16

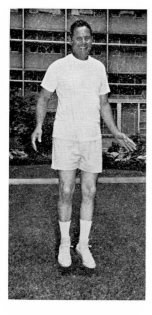

✓FIGURE 14. SMALL JUMPS

The subject jumps vertically about six inches
off the ground landing on the anterior aspect
of the feet.

Week	Repetitions per session	Week	Repetitions per session
1	8	13	20
2	8	14	20
3	12	15	20
4	12	16	20
5	16	17	22
6	16	18	22
7	18	19	22
8	18	20	22
9	20	21	24
10	20	22	24
11	20	23	24
12	20	24	24

Lying on Back Position

√ FIGURE 15. ALTERNATE BENT LEG RAISING

While lying supine, the subject grasps the left knee and flexes the thigh. He then repeats the maneuver with the right knee, completing the cycle.

Week	Repetitions per session	Week	Repetitions per session	Week	Repetitions per session
1	4	9	10	17	12
2	4	10	10	18	12
3	6	11	10	19	12
4	6	12	10	20	12
5	8	13	10	21	14
6	8	14	10	22	14
7	8	15	10	23	14
8	8	16	10	24	14

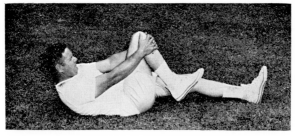

√ FIGURE 16. ALTERNATE STRAIGHT LEG RAISING

While lying supine the subject elevates the left leg to a 45 degree angle with the floor, keeping the knee straight. He repeats this with the right leg, completing one sequence.

Week	Repetitions per session	Week	Repetitions per session	Week	Repetitions per session
1	2	9	8	17	12
2	2	10	8	18	12
3	3	11	10	19	12
4	3	12	10	20	12
5	4	13	10	21	14
6	4	14	10	22	14
7	6	15	10	23	14
8	6	16	10	24	14

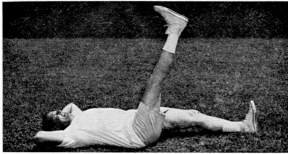

✓ Figure 17. Double Leg Raising and Lowering

While lying supine the subject elevates both legs to a 45 degree angle with the floor, keeping the knees straight.

Week	Repetitions per session	Week	Repetitions per session	Week	Repetitions per session
1	2	9	8	1·7	12
2	2	10	8	18	12
3	3	11	10	19	12
4	3	12	10	20	12
5	4	13	10	21	14
6	4	14	10	22	14
7	6	15	10	23	14
8	6	16	10	24	14

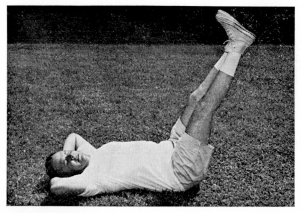

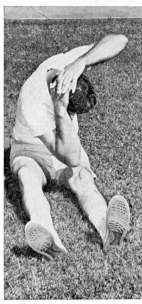

✓ Figure 18. Rocking Situps

While lying supine with hands behind the head, the subject rocks to a sitting position and touches both elbows to the flexed knees.

Week	Repetitions per session	Week	Repetitions per session
1	2	13	10
2	2	14	10
3	3	15	10
4	3	16	10
5	4	17	12
6	4	18	12
7	6	19	12
8	6	20	12
9	8	21	14
10	8	22	14
11	10	23	14
12	10	24	14

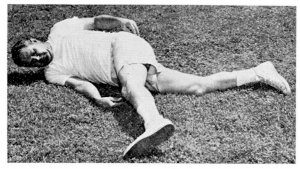

FIGURE 19. LEG CROSSOVER

While lying supine the subject raises the right leg and touches the floor on his left with his toes. He returns to a flat position and completes one cycle by touching his left toes to the floor on his right.

Week	Repetitions per session	Week	Repetitions per session	Week	Repetitions per session
1	1	9	5	17	8
2	1	10	5	18	8
3	2	11	6	19	8
4	2	12	6	20	8
5	3	13	6	21	10
6	3	14	6	22	10
7	4	15	6	23	10
8	4	16	6	24	10

Side Position

FIGURE 20. SIDE LEG RAISES

While lying on the left side the subject raises his right leg as high as he can for the recommended number of repetitions. He then switches to the right side and raises the left leg the same number of times.

Week	Repetitions per session	Week	Repetitions per session	Week	Repetitions per session
1	4	9	10	17	12
2	4	10	10	18	12
3	6	11	10	19	12
4	6	12	10	20	12
5	8	13	10	21	14
6	8	14	10	22	14
7	8	15	10	23	14
8	8	16	10	24	14

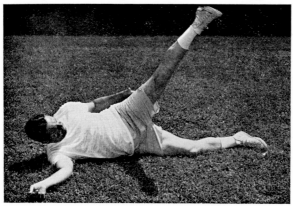

Front (prone) Position

FIGURE 21. CHEST AND LEG RAISING

Assuming a prone position the subject places the arms overhead and raises the upper part of the body and the legs as far off the ground as possible.

Week	Repetitions per session	Week	Repetitions per session	Week	Repetitions per session
1	2	9	10	17	10
2	2	10	10	18	10
3	3	11	10	19	12
4	3	12	10	20	12
5	5	13	10	21	12
6	5	14	10	22	12
7	8	15	10	23	12
8	8	16	10	24	12

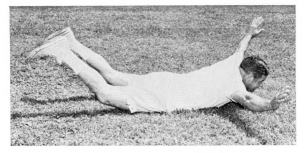

FIGURE 22. KNEE PUSHUPS

The subject positions himself on his hands and knees and touches his chest to the floor.

Week	Repetitions per session	Week	Repetitions per session	Week	Repetitions per session
1	4	9	12	17	14
2	4	10	12	18	14
3	6	11	12	19	16
4	6	12	12	20	16
5	8	13	14	21	16
6	8	14	14	22	16
7	8	15	14	23	16
8	8	16	14	24	16

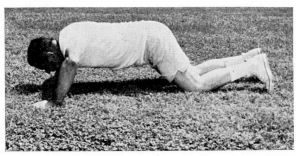

Sitting Position

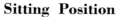

FIGURE 23. TRUNK TWISTING

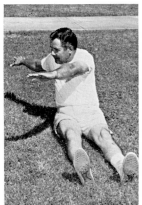

The subject sits with legs out straight and with arms raised to a horizontal position. He twists his trunk to the left, returns to the original position, and completes one sequence by twisting the trunk to the right.

Week	Repetitions per session	Week	Repetitions per session
1	4	13	12
2	4	14	12
3	6	15	12
4	6	16	12
5	8	17	12
6	8	18	12
7	8	19	14
8	8	20	14
9	10	21	14
10	10	22	14
11	10	23	14
12	10	24	14

FIGURE 24. REVERSE PUSHUPS

The subject assumes a sitting position with legs out straight and hands on the floor behind his back. He pushes his body off the floor and then returns to the original position.

Week	Repetitions per session	Week	Repetitions per session	Week	Repetitions per session
1	2	9	6	17	8
2	2	10	6	18	8
3	3	11	6	19	10
4	3	12	6	20	10
5	4	13	8	21	10
6	4	14	8	22	10
7	5	15	8	23	10
8	5	16	8	24	10

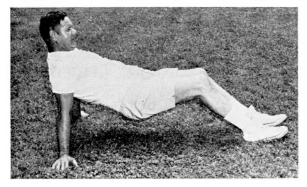

FIGURE 25. REACH AND TOUCH

The subject assumes a sitting position with legs slightly flexed and arms at the sides. He touches the toes with his fingertips and returns to the resting position.

Week	Repetitions per session	Week	Repetitions per session	Week	Repetitions per session
1	4	9	10	17	12
2	4	10	10	18	12
3	6	11	10	19	14
4	6	12	10	20	14
5	8	13	12	21	14
6	8	14	12	22	14
7	8	15	12	23	14
8	8	16	12	24	14

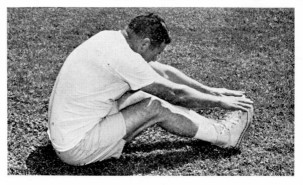

The *walk-jog activity* (Fig. 26) for a given week is described in Table 4. The overall goal is to work up to a one-mile jog after twelve months, during which time the pulse is maintained at 70 percent of predicted maximum heart rate (Fig. 4). A cardiopacer* (Fig. 27) is used initially in the present studies to determine the level of exercise required to maintain this heart rate. The cardiopacer is a battery-driven device which may be carried in a packet or attached to the clothing. A pair of light-weight electrodes are applied to the chest and a small earphone (hearing aid type) is placed in the ear and plugged into the battery device. The cardiopacer is set at the desired exercise heart rate and is switched on when exercise begins. The earphone relates the patient's own heartbeat until the target heart rate is approached, at which time the earphone remains silent as long as the pulse rate remains within a few beats of the desired rate. A warning tone is sounded when the heart rate exceeds the preset rate. Patients can usually be instructed in checking their own pulse rates

*Physiometrics Incorporated
 27727 Pacific Coast Highway
 Malibu, California 90265

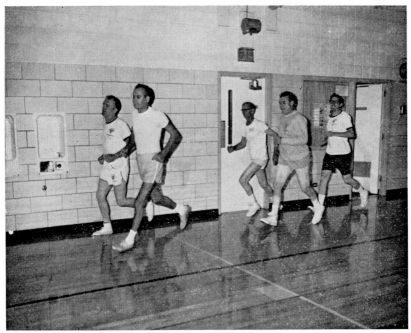

FIGURE 26. Postmyocardial infarction patients engaging in supervised walk-jog activities. (Courtesy of Ervin Miller, Mayo Clinic.)

TABLE 4
CORONARY GROUP WALK AND JOG CHART
PRIOR TO CALISTHENICS
(Perform minimum of 3 times per week)

Week 1 to 4	Walk slowly 100 yards, walk briskly 100 yards, alternately for ¼ mile.
Week 5 to 8	Walk slowly 100 yards, walk briskly 100 yards, alternately ½ mile.
Week 8 to 12	Walk slowly 100 yards, walk briskly 100 yards, jog 100 yards alternately for ½ mile.
Week 13 to 15	Walk briskly 220 yards, jog 220 yards, alternately for ¾ mile.
Week 16 to 24	Jog 440 yards, walk 220 yards, alternately for 1 mile.
Week 25 and over	Jog 1 mile (maintain pulse rate at 70% maximal).
Week 52 and over	Jog 2 miles.

during interrupted jogging sessions and can thereby adjust their jogging pace with a satisfactory degree of accuracy.

The group activity portion is the most enjoyable to the patient but is potentially the most dangerous if noncompetitive rules are not adhered to. Volleyball (Fig. 28) has been highly successful and requires no special skill for enjoyment. Basketball routines such as free

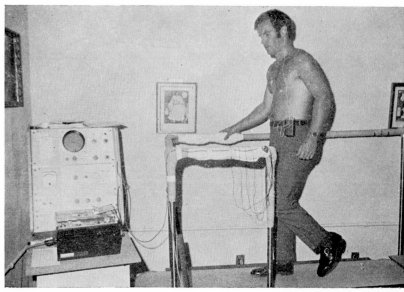

FIGURE 27. A subject demonstrates the use of a cardiopacer. The battery-driven device is seen attached to the subjects belt with lightweight electrode connections applied to the chest wall. A small earphone is plugged into the device. Complete explanation of the use of the cardiopacer is found in the text.

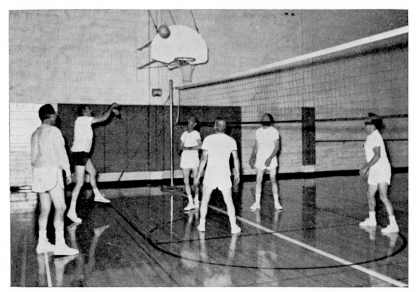

FIGURE 28. Exercise class of patients with coronary heart disease participating in noncompetitive volleyball. (Courtesy of Ervin Miller, Mayo Clinic.)

throws, lay-ups, passing, and full-court dribbling are also well accepted and necessitate almost constant motion. Swimming is a little harder to supervise but is an excellent form of exercise and provides a good change of pace periodically. Indoor hockey is played with a small rubber kickball. The participants are divided into two sides and are equipped with hockey sticks. The object of the game is to advance the ball past a goalie and into the net at each end of the playing surface. The players are not allowed to run and may not leave their feet. No scores are kept, again for the purpose of decreasing the intensity of the workout. In the summer months the patients may exercise outdoors, provided that the resuscitation equipment can be set up nearby. Additional group activities such as bicycle riding and golf practice can be added to the regimen. The dropout rate can be minimized by providing such a wide variety of group activities.

The progress of the exercising coronary patient can be followed in several ways. If a treadmill and equipment for oxygen consumption determination is available, this is used to determine the initial level of fitness and to record changes at two-month intervals. Using the fixed speed treadmill test (Table 1), an expired air sample is collected with a Douglas bag between the fifth and sixth minutes of exercise. The resulting maximal oxygen uptake is recorded in milli-

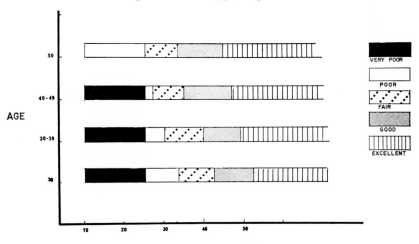

OXYGEN CONSUMPTION (ml/kg/min)

FIGURE 29. Graph showing physical fitness categories based on oxygen consumption and adjusted for age. Adapted from data of K.H. Cooper, M.D. (see text for reference).

liters per kilogram per minute. In general, values below 25 are considered low, those between 30 and 40 average, and those above 40 high (Fig. 29).[111] The average initial value in Hellerstein's study[21] was 23.2 ml/kg/min. This rose to an average of 28.9 ml/kg/min on follow-up testing. Clausen *et al.*[65] noted a similar increase in maximal oxygen uptake in nine patients with coronary disease who exercised regularly over a four to six week period. If a treadmill or bicycle ergometer is not available the bench test measurement of pulse recovery (Fig. 30) is used as a rough index of the conditioning re-

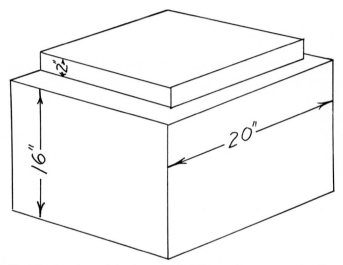

FIGURE 30. The bench used in the modified Harvard step test; the dimensions are specified as seen in Table 5.

sponse,[112] and can be easily repeated at intervals of two months. This test is a modification of the Harvard Step Test. The height of the bench is adjusted according to the patient's height (Table 5). It is preferable to monitor the electrocardiogram during the test in a manner previously described for the treadmill test. The individual steps up and down on the bench at a rate of thirty times per minute for a total of four minutes. At the point of fatigue or upon completion of the test, the patient rests in a chair for one minute and then has pulse rate determinations during the first thirty seconds of each of the following three minutes. The three numbers are added together and a pulse recovery index and fitness grade are assigned according to the scale in Table 5.

TABLE 5
BENCH TEST DETERMINATION OF
POSTEXERCISE PULSE RECOVERY
(See text for details of testing)

Subject Height		Bench Height
5 ft, 3 in to 5 ft, 9 in		16 in
5 ft, 9 in to 6 ft		18 in
over 6 ft		20 in
Total Pulse Counts	*Recovery Index*	*Fitness Grade*
> 198	< 61	Poor
171 to 198	61 to 70	Fair
150 to 170	71 to 80	Good
133 to 149	81 to 90	Very Good
< 133	> 90	Excellent

Abbreviations: ft = feet; in = inches; Total Pulse Count = total number of pulse beats during first 30 seconds of each of the first three minutes following exercise; > Greater; < Less Than.

It is unrealistic to think that all coronary patients can be reconditioned by physical training. Some patients with irreversible mycardial damage secondary to diffuse coronary atherosclerosis occur. If there is no improvement in treadmill performance, maximal oxygen uptake, or pulse recovery (bench test) after six months of phyical training, such individuals probably should be removed from the exercise program as they tend to retard the progress of other group members and increase the risk of a cardiac catastrophe during the exercise sessions. Their removal from the program shoud be done with considerable tact and they should be encouraged to follow a daily walking program, mainly for subjective benefits.

To recapitulate, physical training is a promising new weapon in our armamentarium against coronary heart disease. The program described herein can be modified so that it can be used in a major medical center complete with sophisticated (and expensive) testing devices, or in a relatively small community equipped with only an interested physician and patient. To further illustrate the chamelion-like nature of this program, let us consider the following two cases:

Case 1

A 42-year-old man made an uneventful recovery from a myocardial infarction and five months later consulted his internist about physical activity. He was referred to the nearby university medical center where he underwent a complete physical examination, which included having the following laboratory tests: electrocardiogram, chest x-ray, serum cholesterol and triglycerides, two hour postprandial blood sugar, vital capacity, MMPI, and skin-fold measurements. On initial treadmill testing he progressed only to the third level, stopping because of generalized fatigue. His maximal oxygen uptake was low, being 19 ml/kg/min. He was enrolled in the previously described exercise program and progressed according to schedule for the first eight weeks, experiencing no adverse musculoskeletal side effects. Repeat testing revealed that he was able to complete the fourth level of treadmill elevation. The oxygen uptake was now 24 ml/kg/min. As he began the ninth week of exercise, a cardiopacer was used to regulate his jogging pace at that necessary to maintain a pulse rate of 135 beats/min. This pace was well tolerated by the patient. Radio-telemetry revealed no S-T segment depression or arrthymias.

Case 2

A 49-year-old man had been admitted to a small community hospital (eighty beds) for evaluation of severe angina pectoris. His physical examination was unremarkable, and there were no abnormalities in serum lipids or in glucose tolerance. He was advised to stop cigarette smoking and was started on a combination of isosorbide dinitrate and propranolol. Despite maximum doses of the latter he continued to require an average of fifteen nitroglycerine tablets daily and was unable to hold a job. Coronary arteriograms revealed a 75 percent narrowing of the left anterior descending coronary artery and a 60 percent occlusion of the right circumflex coronary. The patient was enrolled in a physical training program at the local YMCA. The group was small, numbering only four men and was supervised by a physical director and a physician. Initially he was given a Masters test (which was positive) and found to have a pulse recovery index (Table 5) of 60, which was poor. Although initially quite apprehensive during the exercise sessions, he had no difficulty in following the weekly exercise prescription. At two-month intervals he had follow-up Masters two-step and pulse recovery testing; the former remained positive, although the S-T segment depression was reduced from 2 to 1 mm, while the pulse recovery index was now 75, which was indicative of a good response. With a little practice the patient was able to measure his radial pulse rate during interrupted jogging and adjusted his pace to maintain an average pulse rate of 130 beats/min. He was able to return to work but still required approximately five nitroglycerine tablets per day.

VIII

SUMMARY

I N THIS BOOK we have attempted to review and discuss the somewhat controversial issue of exercise and coronary heart disease and have covered historical aspects as well as a discussion of the advantages and disadvantages. It is felt that the use of exercise in the proper manner will utilize the advantages and tend to eliminate the disadvantages, complications and risks. In dealing with exercise we feel that it can be made proper by recommending the use of those types of physical activity that affect and increase the work (myocardial oxygen consumption) of the heart, thus tending to condition (train) the patient to the point at which he can obtain higher levels of physical activity without further increasing the work of the heart.

We have also emphasized the value of exercise testing of patients to determine the heart rate and blood pressure response to certain levels of exercise in order to recommend the safest and best level of exercise for their physical conditioning; in addition, we recommend this for detection of arrhythmias and ischemic S-T segment changes.

Lastly, we have commented on the issue of proper exercise in the alteration of risk factors; additional well-controlled studies are needed. This is particularly true in view of the International Cooperative Study on Cardiovascular Epidemiology, which did not show a clear association between coronary proneness and physical inactivity.[56] In an editorial comment on the latter results, Paul correctly states that "this is surely a complex issue, and from this kind of evidence the value of physical exercise in coronary disease prevention should neither be readily dismissed nor be adopted with evangelistic fervor as some have."[113] We favor a common sense approach to exercise prescription, recognizing that controlled studies are nonexistent in this area. Exercise is inexpensive, enjoyable to most and so far appears safe

[49]

for the coronary-prone individual if done properly. The latter necessitates thorough preliminary evaluation and medical supervision. If the only beneficial effect of exercise in the coronary patient was an alleviation of fear, anxiety and sense of impending doom, that alone would validate the time and cost of research in this area to date.

REFERENCES

1. Enos, W.F., Holmes, R.H., and Beyer, J.: Coronary disease among United States soldiers killed in action in Korea. *JAMA, 152*:1090-1093, 1953.

2. Mason, J.K.: Asymptomatic disease of coronary arteries in young men. *Brit Med J, 2*:1234-1237, 1963.

3. Viel, B., Donoso, S., and Salcedo, D.: Coronary atherosclerosis in persons dying violently. *Arch Intern Med (Chicago), 122*:97-103, 1968.

4. Fox, S.M., and Skinner, J.S.: Physical activity and cardiovascular health. *Amer J Cardiol, 14*:731-746, 1964.

5. Parmley, L.F.: Proceedings of the National Conference on exercise in the prevention, in the evaluation, in the treatment of heart disease. *J S Carolina Med Ass, 65*:i, 1969.

6. Alexander, J.K.: Exercise and coronary heart disease. *Cardiovasc Res Cent Bull* (Baylor College of Medicine), *8*:2-7, 1969.

7. Paul Dudley White: Personal communication, September, 1969.

8. Currens, J.H., and White, P.D.: Half a century of running: Clinical, physiological and autopsy findings in the case of Clarence DeMar, ("Mr. Marathon"). *New Eng J Med, 265*:988-993, 1961.

9. Katz, L.N., and Miller, A.J.: Physical activity and coronary heart disease. *Hosp Med,* :63-66, 1968.

10. Morris, J.N., Heady, J.A., Raffle, P.A.B., Roberts, C.G., and Parks, J.W.: Coronary heart disease and physical activity of work. *Lancet, 2*:1053-1057, 1953.

11. Fox, S.M., and Paul, O.: Physical activity and coronary heart disease. *Amer J Cardiol, 23*:298-303, 1969.

12. Morris, J.N., and Crawford, M.D.: Coronary heart disease and physical activity at work. *Brit Med J, 2*:1485, 1958.

13. Breslow, L., and Buell, P.: Mortality from coronary heart disease and physical activity of work in California. *J Chronic Dis, 11*:421-444, 1960.

14. Frank, C.W., Weinblatt, E., Shapiro, S., and Sager, R.V.: Physical inactivity as a lethal factor in myocardial infarction among men. *Circulation, 34*:1022-1033, 1964.

15. Eckstein, R.W.: Effect of exercise and coronary artery narrowing on coronary collateral circulation. *Cir Res, 5*:230-235, 1957.

16. Tepperman, J., and Pearlman, D.: Effects of exercise and anemia on coronary arteries of small animals as revealed by the corrosion-cast technique. *Circ Res, 9*:576-584, 1961.

17. Stevenson, J.A.F., Feleki, V., Rechnitzer, P., and Beaton, J.R.: Effect of exercise on coronary tree size in the rat. *Circ Res, 15*:265, 1964.
18. Kaplinsky, E., Hood, W.B., Jr., McCarthy, B., McCombs, H.L., and Lown, B.: Effects of physical training in dogs with coronary artery ligation. *Circulation, 37*:556-565, 1968.
19. Kattus, A.A., Jr., Hanafee, W.N., Longmire, W.P., Jr., MacAlpin, R.N., and Rivin, A.U.: Diagnostic, medical and surgical management of coronary insufficiency. *Ann Intern Med, 69*:115-136, 1968.
20. Frick, M.H.: The effect of physical training in manifest ischemic heart disease. *Circulation, 40*:433-435, 1969.
21. Hellerstein, H.K.: Exercise therapy in coronary disease. *Bull NY Acad Med, 44*:1028-1047, 1968.
22. Spiekerman, R.: Personal communication, March, 1970.
23. Keys, A., Arovanis, C., Blackburn, H.W. *et al.*: Epidemiological studies related to coronary heart disease: Characteristics of men aged 40-59 in seven countries. *Acta Med Scand Suppl, 460*:1, 1966.
24. Stamler, J., Kjelsfurg, M., and Hall Y.: Epidemiologic studies on cardio-vascular-renal disease. *J Chronic Dis, 12*:440-475, 1960.
25. Cantwell, J.D., and Fletcher, G.F.: Cardiac complications while jogging. *JAMA, 210*:130-131, 1969.
26. Harris, W.E., Bowerman, W., McFadden, R.B., and Kerns, T.A.: Jogging. An adult exercise program. *JAMA, 201*:759-761, 1967.
27. Cohen, H.J.: Jogger's petechiae. *New Eng J Med, 279*:109, 1968.
28. Seigel, I.M.: Jogger's heel. *JAMA, 206*:2899, 1968.
29. Hunder, G.G.: Harmful effects of jogging. *Ann Intern Med, 71*:664-665, 1969.
30. Mann, G.V., Garrett, H.L., Farhi, A., Murray, H., and Billings, F.T.: Exercise to prevent coronary heart disease. An experimental study of the effects of training on risk factors for coronary disease in men. *Amer J Med, 46*:12-27, 1969.
31. Fletcher, G.F.: Exercise and the heart. *Access, 2* (No. 5), 1970.
32. Falls, H.B.: Proceedings of the National Conference on Exercise in the prevention, in the evaluation and in the treatment of heart disease. The relative energy requirements of various physical activities in relation to physiological strain. *J S Carolina Med Ass, 65*:8, 1969.
33. Wells, J.G., Balke, B., and Van Fossan, D.D.: Lactic acid accumulation during work; a suggested standardization of work classification. *J Appl Physiol, 10*:51-55, 1957.
34. Sarnoff, S.J., Braunwald, E., Welch, G.F., Jr., Case, R.B., Stainsby, W.N., and Machruz, R.: Hemodynamic determinants of oxygen consumption of the heart with special reference to the tension time index. *Amer J Physiol, 192*:148-156, 1958.

35. Monroe, R.G., and Frence, G.N.: Left ventricular pressure-volume relationships and myocardial oxygen consumption in the isolated heart. *Cir Res, 9*:362-374, 1961.

36. Robinson, B.F.: Relation of heart rate and systolic blood pressure to the onset of pain in angina pectoris. *Circulation, 35*:1073-1083, 1967.

37. Mitchell, J.H., Sproule, B.J., and Chapman, C.B.: The physiological meaning of the maximal oxygen intake test. *J Clin Invest, 37*:538-547, 1958.

38. Frick, M.H., Konttinen, A., and Sarajas, H.S.S.: Effects of physical training on circulation at rest and during exercise. *Amer J. Cardiol, 12*: 142-147, 1963.

39. Saltin, B., Blomquist, G., Mitchell, J.H., Johnson, R.L., Jr., Wildenthal, K., and Chapman, C.B.: Response to exercise after bed rest and after training. *Circulation, 38 (Supp VII)*: 1-78, 1968.

40. Siegel, W., Blomqvist, G., and Mitchell, J.H.: Effects of a quantitated physical training program on middle-aged sedentary men. *Circulation, 41*:19-29, 1970.

41. Grimby, G., and Salton, B.: Physiological analysis of physically well trained middle-aged and old athletes. *Acta Med Scand, 179*:513, 1966.

42. Naughton, J., Shanbour, K., Armstrong, R., McCoy, J., and Lategola, M.T.: Cardiovascular responses to exercise following myocardial infarction. *Arch Intern Med (Chicago), 117*:541-545, 1966.

43. Varnauskas, E., Bergman, H., Houk, P., and Bjorntorp, P.: Hemodynamic effects of physical training in coronary patients. *Lancet, 2*:8-12, 1966.

44. Frick, M.H., and Katila, M.: Hemodynamic consequences of physical training after myocardial infarction. *Circulation, 37*:192-202, 1968.

45. Sheffield, L.T., Roitman, D., and Reeves, T.J.: Submaximal exercise testing. *J S Carolina Med Ass, 65*:18-25, 1969.

46. Frick, M.H., Elovainic, R.O., and Somer, T.: The mechanism of bradycardia evoked by physical training. *Cardiologia (Basel), 51*:46-54, 1967.

47. Master, A.M., and Oppenheimer, E.R.: A simple exercise tolerance test for circulatory efficiency with standard tables for normal individuals. *Amer J Med Sci, 177*:223, 1929.

48. Doan, A.E., Peterson, D.R., Blackmon, J.R., and Bruce, R.A.: Myocardial ischemia after maximal exercise in healthy men. A method for detecting potential coronary heart disease? *Amer Heart J, 69*:11-21, 1965.

49. Doyle, J.T., Heslin, A.S., Hilliboe, H.E., Formel, P.F., and Korns, R.F.: A prospective study of degenerative cardiovascular disease in Albany: Report of three years' experience—Ischemic heart disease. Symposium —Measuring the risk of coronary heart disease in adult population groups. *Amer J Public Health, 47 (Part 2)*:25, April 1957.

50. Roitman, D., Jones, W.B., and Sheffield, L.T.: Comparison of submaximal

exercise ECG test with coronary cineangiocardiogram. *Ann Intern Med, 72*:641-647, 1970.

51. Dawber, T.R., and Kannel, W.B.: Susceptibility to coronary heart disease. *Mod Conc Cardiovasc Dis, 30*:671-676, 1961.

52. Doyle, J.T.: Etiology of coronary disease: Risk factors influencing coronary disease. *Mod Conc Cardiovasc Dis, 35*:81-86, 1966.

53. Stamler, J., Berkson, D.M., Lindberg, H.A., *et al.*: Coronary risk factors: Their impact, and their therapy in the prevention of coronary heart disease. *Med Clin N Amer, 50*:229-254, 1966.

54. Ostrander, L.D., Jr.: Alterations of factors predisposing to coronary heart disease. *Ann Intern Med, 68*:1072-1077, 1968.

55. Rosenman, R.H., Friedman, M., Straus, R., Wurm, M., Kositchek, R., Hahn, W., and Werthesse, N.T.: A predictive study of coronary heart disease. The Western Collaborative Group Study. *JAMA, 189*:15-22, 1964.

56. Keys, A.: Coronary heart disease in seven countries. *Circulation 41 (Suppl. 1)*:1-198, 1970.

57. Trulson, M.F., Clancy, R.E., Jessop, W.J.E., Childers, R.W., and Stare, F.J.: Comparisons of siblings in Boston and Ireland. *J Amer Diet Ass, 45*:225, 1964.

58. Mann, G.V., Shaffer, R.D., and Rick, A.: Physical fitness and immunity to heart disease in masai. *Lancet, 2*:1308-1310, 1965.

59. Shaper, A.G., and Jones, K.W.: Serum-cholesterol in camel-herding nomads. *Lancet, 2*:1305-1307, 1962.

60. Cantwell, J.D.: Coronary heart disease in young prisoners. In preparation.

61. Walker, W.J., and Gregoratos, G.: Myocardial infarction in young men. *Amer J. Cardiol, 19*:339-343, 1967.

62. Fredrickson, D.S., Levy, R.I., and Lees, R.S.: Fat transport in lipoproteins —an intergrated approach to mechanisms and disorders. *New Eng J Med, 276*:34-44,94-103,148-156,215-224,273-281, 1967.

63. Dalderup, L.M., DeVoogd, N., Meyknecht, E.A., *et al.*: The effects of increasing the daily physical activity on the serum cholesterol levels. *Nutr Dieta (Basel), 9*:112-123, 1967.

64. Hoffman, A.A., Nelson, W.R., and Goss, F.A.: Effects of an exercise program on plasma lipids of senior Air Force officers. *Amer J Cardiol, 20*:516-524, 1967.

65. Clausen, J.P., Larse, O.A., and Trap-Jensen, J.: Physical training in the management of coronary artery disease. *Circulation, 40*:143-154, 1969.

66. Hellerstein, H.K.: The effects of physical activity: Patients and normal coronary prone subjects. *Minn Med, 52*:1335-1341, 1969.

67. Calvy, G.L., Cady, L.D., Mufson, M.A., Nierman, B.A., and Gertler, M.M.: Serum lipids and enzymes. Their levels after high-caloric, high-fat intake and vigorous exercise regimen in Marine Corps recruit personnel. *JAMA, 183*:1-4, 1963.

68. Holloszy, J.O., Skinner, J.S., Toto, G., and Cureton, T.K.: Effects of a six month program of endurance exercise on the serum lipids of middle-aged men. *Amer J Cardiol, 14*:753-760, 1964.

69. Golding, L.A.: Effects of physical training upon total serum cholesterol levels. *Res Quart Amer Ass Health Phys Educ, 32*:499, 1961.

70. Stanley, E., and Kezdi, P.: Training variations in middle-aged males. *Circulation, 38 (Suppl. VI)*:189, 1968.

71. Karvonen, M.W.: Effects of vigorous exercise on the heart. In Rosenbaum, F.F., and Belknap, E. (Eds.): *Work and the Heart.* New York, Paul B Hoebner, Inc. 1959, p. 190.

72. Rochelle, R.: Blood plasma cholesterol changes during a physical training program. *Res Quart Amer Ass Health Phys Educ, 32*:538, 1961.

73. Romanova, D., and Barbarin, P.: The influence of physical exercises on the content of serum protein, lipoprotein and total cholesterol in persons of middle and elderly age with symptoms of atherosclerosis. *Kardiologiia, 1*:36, 1961.

74. Mirkin, G.: Labile serum cholesterol values. *New Eng J Med, 279*:1001, 1968.

75. Nikkila, E.A., and Konttinen, A.: Effect of physical activity on postprandial levels of fats in serum. *Lancet, 1*:1151-1154, 1962.

76. Cohen, H., and Goldberg, C.: Effects of physical exercise on alimentary lipemia. *Brit Med J, 2*:509-511, 1960.

77. Goode, R.C., Firstbrook, J.B., and Shephard, R.J.: Effects of exercise and cholesterol—free diet on human serum lipids. *Canad J Physiol Pharmacol, 44*:575-580, 1966.

78. Miall, W.E., and Oldham, P.D.: Factors influencing arterial blood pressure in the general population. *Clin Sci, 17*:409-444, 1958.

79. Kapeller-She, A.M.: Prehypertensive state in residents of Peking. *Fed Proc, 22*:T-778-781, 1963.

80. Boyer, J.L., and Kasch, F.W.: Exercise therapy in hypertensive men. *JAMA, 211*:1668-1671, 1970.

81. Mellerowicz, H.: Vergleichende Untersuchungen über das Öknomieprinvip in Arbeit und Leistung des trainierten Kreislaufs und seine Bedeutung für die präventive und rehabilitive Medizi. *Arch Kreislaufforsch, 24*:70, 1956.

82. Levine, S.A., Gordon, B., and Derick, C.L.: Some changes in the chemical constituents of the blood following a marathon race with special reference to the development of hypoglycemia. *JAMA, 82*:1778-1779, 1924.

83. Blotner, H.: Effect of prolonged physical inactivity on tolerance of sugar. *Arch Intern Med (Chicago), 75*:39-44, 1945.

84. Davidson, P.C., Shane, S.R., and Albrink, M.J.: Decreased glucose tolerance following a physical conditioning program. *Circulation, 7*:(*Suppl. III*) 1966.

85. Skinner, J.S., Holloszy, J.O., and Cureton, T.K.: Effects of a program of

endurance exercises on physical work. *Amer J. Cardiol, 14*:747-752, 1964.

86. Rechnitzer, P.A., Yuhasz, M.S., Paivio, A., Pickard, H.A., and Lefcoe, N.: Effects of a 24-week exercise programme on normal adults and patients with previous myocardial infarction. *Brit Med J, 1*:734-735, 1967.

87. McPherson, B.D., Paivo, A., Yuhasz, M.S., Rechnitzer, P.A., Pickard, H.A., and Lefcoe, N.M.: Psychological effects of an exercise program for post-infarction and normal adult men. *J Sports Med, 7*:3, 1967.

88. Naughton, J., Bruhn, J.G., and Lategola, M.T.: Effects of physical training on physiological and behavioral characteristics of cardiac patients. *Arch Phys Med, 49*:131, 1968.

89. Hellerstein, H.K., and Friedman, E.H.: Sexual activity and the post-coronary patient. *Medical Aspects of Human Sexual, 3*:70, 1969.

90. Hellerstein, H.K., and Friedman, E.H.: Sexual activity and the post-coronary patient. *Arch Intern Med, (Chicago), 125*:987-999, 1970.

91. Baekeland, F.: Exercise deprivation. *Arch Gen Psychiat (Chicago), 22*: 365-369, 1970.

92. Chiang, B.N., Perlman, L.V., Ostrander, L.D., and Epstein, F.H.: Relationship of premature systoles to coronary heart disease and sudden death in the Tecumseh epidemiologic studies. *Ann Intern Med, 70*: 1159-1166, 1969.

93. Kannel, W.B., Gordon, T., Castelli, W.P., and Margolis, J.R.: Electrocardiographic left ventricular hypertrophy and risk of coronary heart disease. *Ann Intern Med, 72*:813-822, 1970.

94. Smith, W.G., Cullen, K.J., and Thorbun, I.O.: Electrocardiograms of marathon runners in 1962 Commonwealth games. *Brit Heart J, 26*: 469-476, 1964.

95. Spann, J.F., Jr., Mason, D.T., and Zelis, R.F.: Recent advances in the understanding of congestive heart failure (II). *Mod Conc Cardiovasc Dis, 39*:79-84, 1970.

96. Hellerstein, H.K., Hirsch, E.Z., Cumber, W., Allen, L., Polster, S., and Zucker, N.: Reconditioning of the coronary patient: A preliminary report. In Likoff, W., and Moyer, J.H. (Eds.): *Coronary Heart Disease.* New York: Grune & Stratton, 1963, p. 448-454.

97. Iatridis, S.G., and Ferguson, J.H.: Effect of physical exercise on blood clotting and fibrinolysis. *J Appl Physiol, 18*:337-344, 1963.

98. Egeberg, O.: The effect of exercise on the blood clotting system. *Scand J Clin Lab Invest, 15*:8-13, 1963.

99. McDonald, G.A., and Fullerton, H.W.: Comparison of animal and vegetable fats in increasing blood coagulability. *Lancet, 2*:598-599, 1958.

100. Guest, M.M., and Celander, D.R.: Fibrinolytic activity in exercise. *Physiologist, 3*:69, 1960.

101. Buzina, R., and Keys, A.: Blood coagulation after a fat meal. *Circulation, 14*:854-858, 1956.

102. McDonald, L., and Edgill, M.: Coagulability of the blood in ischemic heart disease. *Lancet, 2*:457-460, 1957.
103. Montoye, H.J., Howard, G.E., and Wood, J.H.: Observations of some hemochemical and anthropometric measurements in athletes. *J Sports Med, 7*:35-44, 1967.
104. Bosco, J.S., Greenleaf, J.E., Kaye, R.L., and Averkin, E.G.: Reduction of serum uric acid in young men during physical training. *Amer J Cardiol, 25*:46-52, 1970.
105. Dawber, T.R.: Identification of excess cardiovascular risk. A practical approach. *Minn Med, 52*:1217-1221, 1969.
106. Rechnitzer, P.A., Yuhasz, M.S., Pickard, H.A., and Lefcoe, N.M.: The effects of a graduated exercise program on patients with previous myocardial infarction. *Canad Med Ass J, 92*:858-860, 1965.
107. Bass, H., Whitcomb, J.F., and Forman, R.: Exercise training: Therapy for patients with chronic obstructive pulmonary disease. *Chest, 57*: 116-121, 1970.
108. Heberden, W.: Some accounts of a disorder of the breast. *Med Trans Roy Coll Physicians, 2*:59, 1772.
109. Parry, C.H.: *An Inquiry into the Symptoms and Causes of the Syncope Anginosa, Commonly Called Angina Pectoris.* London, Cadell and Davies, 1799, p.148.
110. Gottheimer, V.: Long range strenuous sports training for cardiac reconditioning and rehabilitation. *Amer J Cardiol, 22*:426-435, 1968.
111. Cooper, K.H.: *The New Aerobics.* New York, Evans and Co., 1970, p. 28.
112. Gallagher, J.R., Allman, F.L., Jr., Guild, W.R., *et al.*: Is your patient fit? A simple supplementary test for evaluating a patients fitness. *JAMA, 201*:117-118, 1967.
113. Paul, O.: The international cooperative study on epidemiology. *Circulation, 41*:895-897, 1970.